WATER RUNNING

DOWNHILL!

WATER RUNNING

DOWNHILL!

WORDS OF EMPOWERMENT
FOR WOMEN IN MIDLIFE

BY:

JOAN ELLEN GAGE

iUniverse, Inc.
New York Lincoln Shanghai

WATER RUNNING DOWNHILL!
WORDS OF EMPOWERMENT FOR WOMEN IN MIDLIFE

iUniverse books may be ordered through booksellers or by contacting:

iUniverse
2021 Pine Lake Road, Suite 100
Lincoln, NE 68512
www.iuniverse.com
1-800-Authors (1-800-288-4677)

Because of the dynamic nature of the Internet, any Web addresses or links contained in this book may have changed since publication and may no longer be valid.

The views expressed in this work are solely those of the author and do not necessarily reflect the views of the publisher, and the publisher hereby disclaims any responsibility for them.

ISBN: 978-0-595-42545-7 (pbk)
ISBN: 978-0-595-86873-5 (ebk)

Printed in the United States of America

This book is dedicated to all of the *girl gang*. We have shared each other's losses and triumphs, tears and laughter. We are all sisters, but sisters of *__choice__*.

"Feel the fear and do it anyway."

—*Susan Jeffers*

Contents

ACKNOWLEDGEMENTS

Thank you all of my friends for being a sounding board for this book. I want to thank my friend and sister Karen, and friends Cyndi, Elisa, Julie, Marion, and Sanja. You have given me unconditional support, and have helped push me out of my nest. Thanks for believing in me!

I especially want to thank my husband, Rob, for his patience, and for being there for me. I thank him for listening, even though he did not understand my ramblings much of the time!

And a special thank you to my Mom and Dad for your faith in me!

INTRODUCTION

These days there is a plethora of information out there for the middle-lifer, especially for women. In my personal approach to mid-life, I have felt like a hang-glider preparing to jump off of a cliff. Some inner force has been guiding and prodding me, as I get nearer and nearer to the edge!

With the publishing of this book I am airborne! I may crash, but I have to try to launch *Water Running Downhill!* I hope that the book brings you inspiration, and laughter. Please share *Water Running Downhill!* with your friends and fly!

WATER RUNNING DOWNHILL!

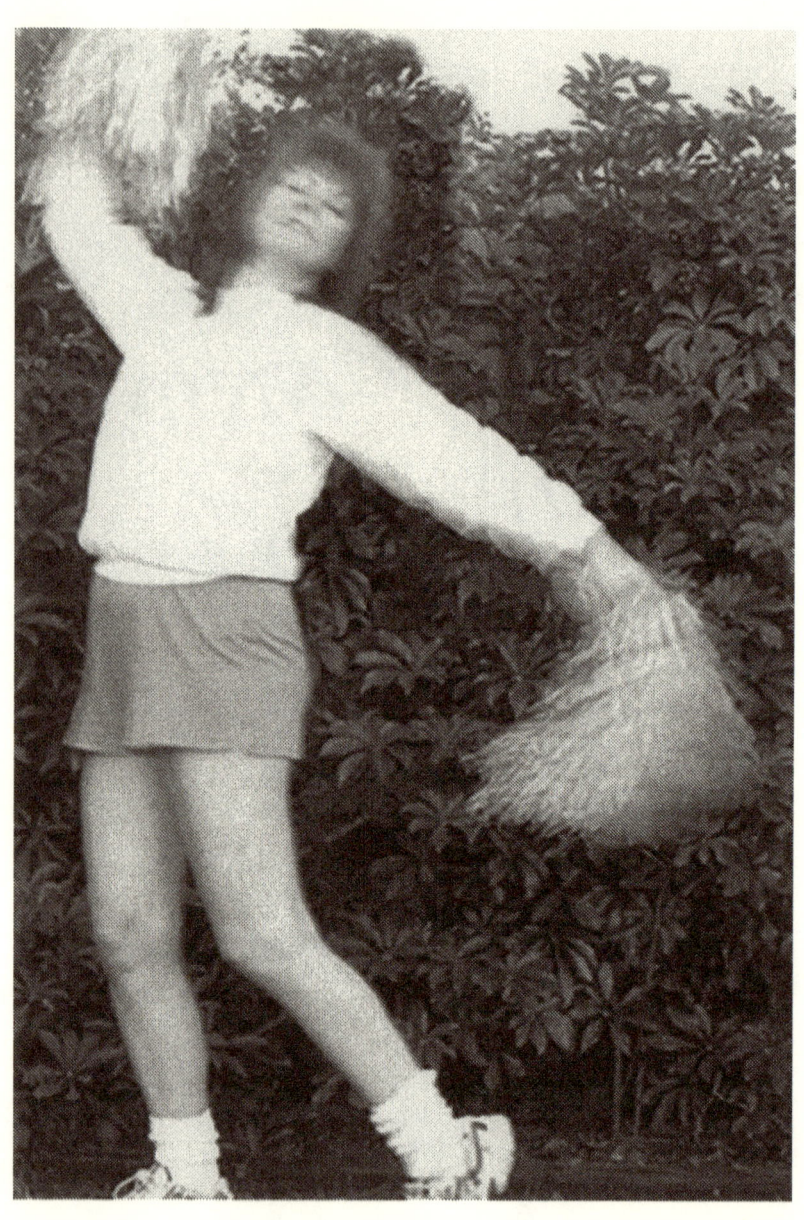

"SIS" BOOM BAH

I am your midlife cheerleader
So chant this cheer out loud
And sing it out with feeling
To make your sisters proud!

Be good to yourselves
Because no one else will
Take time to nurture
You're not over the hill!

Become the balance
Quit the balancing act
Life's passing you by
And you know that's a fact!

Leave office work at work
Remember you exist
You can't have too much fun
So put it on your list!

USED GOODS

There are no
Guarantees or refunds
And no exchanges
You have to take it
As it is

A slight modification
May be possible
But, beyond that
What you see is
What you get

There may be
Surface imperfections
Due to materials used
And the contents
May have settled
During handling

But each piece is
An individually crafted
Unique work of art
A truly one of a kind
Human being

WOMEN

Sisters
Singers of
Sad songs
Seductresses
Strong
Saintly
Soaring
Sage
Sphinxes

Women

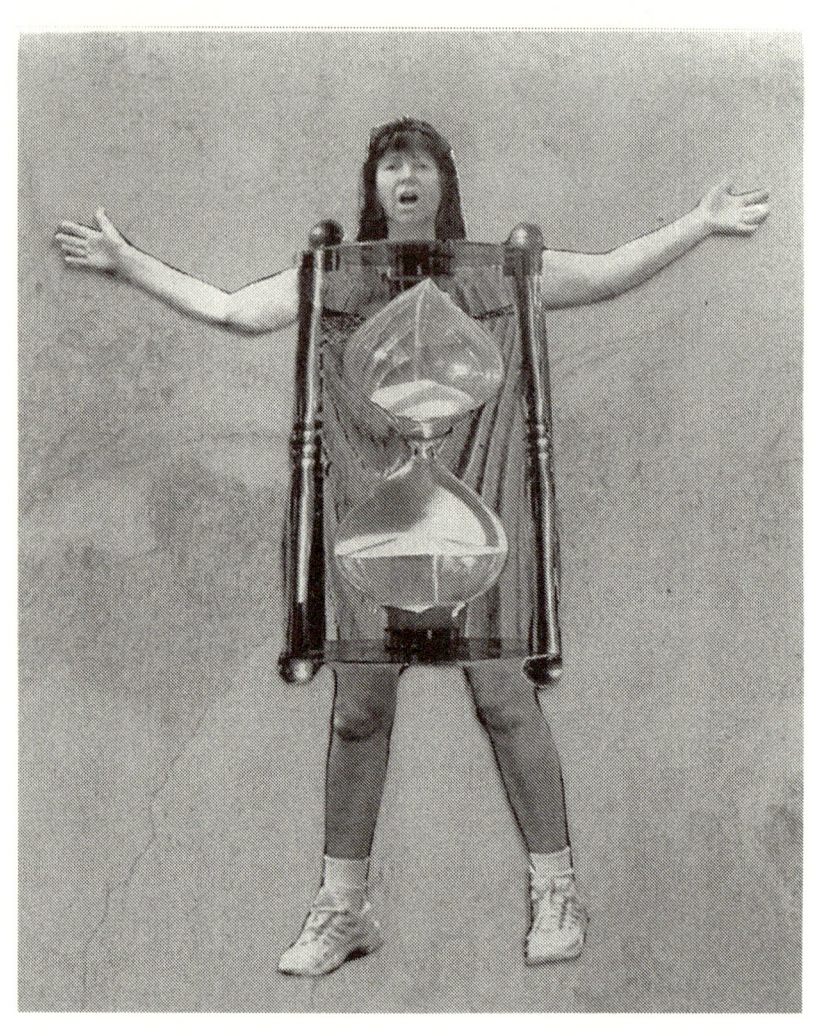

MIDLIFE CLOCK

Time
Too much, not enough
Too slow, too fast
Forever tick, tick, ticking
Away …

Time
We wish it
Here …
We wish it
Gone …

Time
Feel it
Trickling, teasing
Through your fingers
Sifting between
Your toes …

You
Are the hourglass
Your time is running
Out, tick … tock …
Half of the sand
Of your being
Has dwindled away

Your vital force
Diminishes as
Grain by
Tiny grain
Your essence
Erodes …

Wake up
It's half past
Your life!

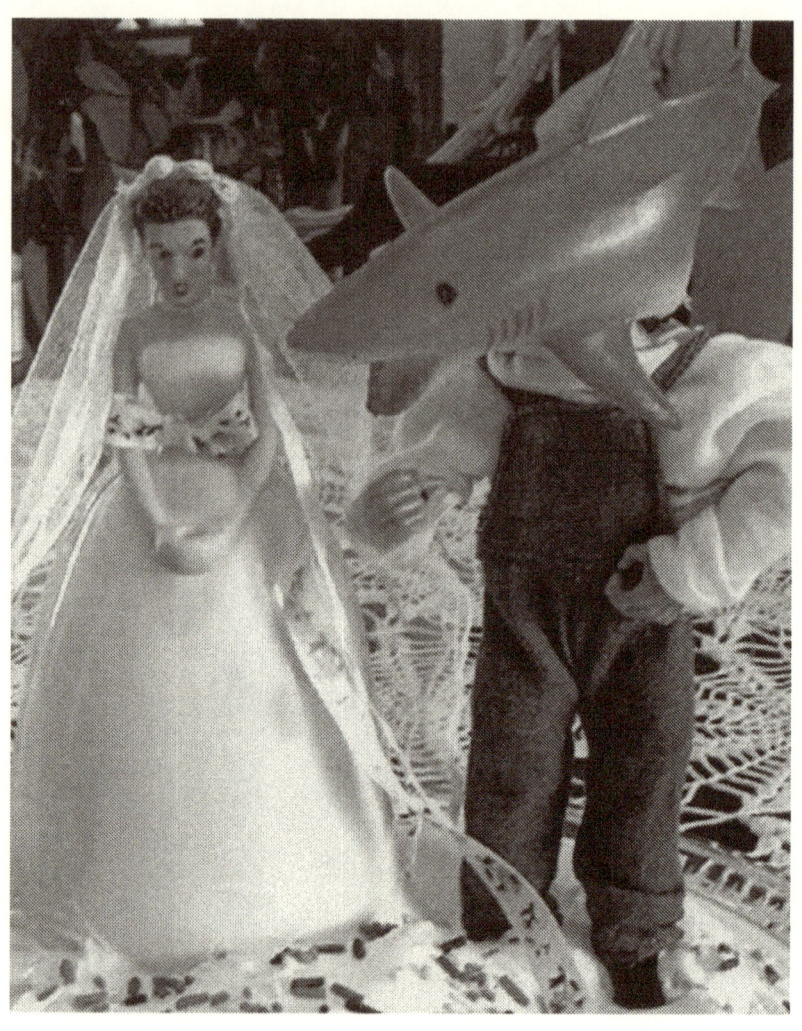

GREAT EXPECTATIONS

We all grew up with the Great American Dream
Expecting to be beautiful and rich
Expecting to marry Prince Charming
Having been breast-fed on fairy tales, and
Brainwashed by happy endings

But, many of us have been disillusioned
Perhaps having gotten pretty (or passable)
And middle classed instead
(If you were lucky)

Prince Charming turned into
Your classic balding
Couch potato, sports-nut
(If you were lucky?)

Possibly, you lost out on the whole enchilada
Marriage, house in the suburbs, 1.5 children
Maybe you're still looking for that perfect love
(Looking to get lucky)

With the worst scenario
You got the Great American Nightmare
Instead
(Whoops! Out of luck)

IF TRUTH BE BOLD

After reaching this
Banner year of years
With much preparation and
Soul searching
What have I learned?

That the experience of
Living continues on
Nothing ends that does
Not set something else
Into motion.

That the erudition is
An on-going and
Ever-changing dynamic where
One must be
Consciously open-minded.

That the universe's mysteries and
Her divine secrets
May remain inscrutable while
They are subject to
Individual interpretation.

That each one makes
Their own happiness
That life's aging shadow
Is ever lengthening.

That one *must* love.

WOOMAN

Women carry a heavy
Burden
Many of us balance
Outside employment and
Home (more work!)
Maybe child rearing completes
The load, all done at the expense of
Self

We juggle our universe while
Multi-tasking, cooking
Car-pooling, shopping
Laundering, errand running
Homework instructing
House cleaning, gardening
Etcetera, etcetera

And get this:
Society dictates that
We maintain our savvy and our good looks
During these amazing feats
(We usually pull this off!)
And, amazingly enough
We are still expected to have
Sex, be sexy, **_and_** stay awake

Ironically,
Even though we function
On a daily basis
As CEO's and their staff
We still can't have
A woman President yet
Go figure?

FOOTFALLS

Women must walk
A different path
Than men
We must walk it
Carefully and
Cautiously
For fear of
Discovery and/or
Criticism

Our paths
Take us to
Alternative planes
Of consciousness
They lead us to the
Oft unexplored territory
Of our minds eye
They bring us to truth
And to sagacity

Choose
And make
The journey unto
Your soul's threshold
Dare
To cross over
To the land of imagination
And your heart of
Creativity

Live
Love life
Morph
Into enlightenment

NEW YEAR'S RESOLUTIONS

We have a new year
They seem to be arriving
At lightening speed
In this new decade

Think of this year as
An opportunity
To grow and celebrate
Toast the women you have become

Forget the past mistakes and
Focus on what makes you
Content and joyous
Be your own best friend

Live life now, not later
For later may not
Be here for you

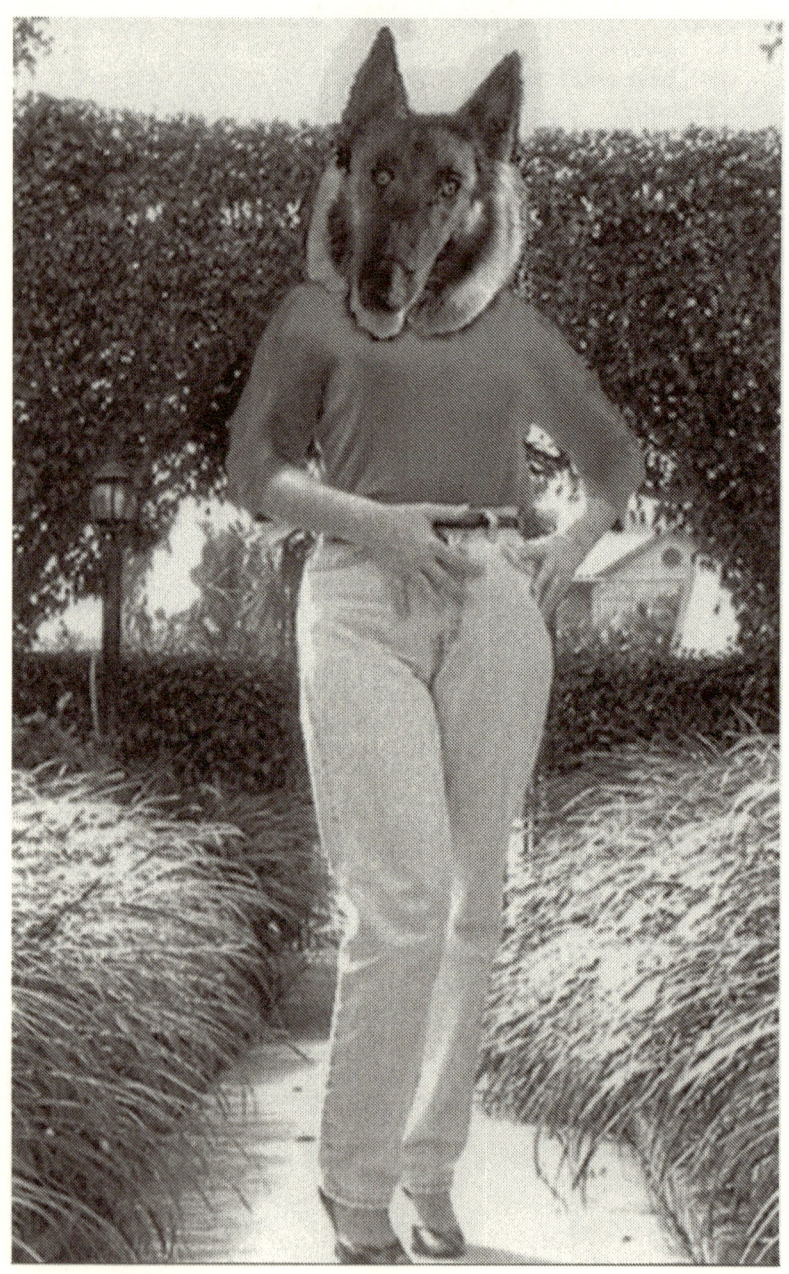

EIGHT IN DOG YEARS (AKA FIFTY!)

Here I am
Stuck
In the middle
Of me

Trying to redefine
My identity
At the precipice of
Midlife, i.e.
Menopause

There
I've said it
The "M" word
(Sounding the death knell
Of youthfulness, as we know it!)

Enter the curse of middle age
See …
Skin sag, lines deepen
Into the antithesis
Of "perky"

Zombies, recite the litany:
"I'm not getting older
I'm getting better"
The Golden Years
(Such rubbish)

Forget that tired rhetoric
News flash! We are supposed to age
We are not Barbie dolls
We are *people*
Let's not fear our natural metamorphosis
May we embrace who we are and
Who we are becoming, with fortitude
We are powerful; we are *WOMEN!*

MENSES SCHMENSES

Mad
Madding
Madness
Mid
Middle
Middling
Moody
Moods

HONEY DO LIST

In menopause will we
Ignore laws
Break jaws
Call our Maws
Pursue a lost cause
Draw straws
Grow moss
Buy gewgaws
Reflect and pause
Make crow caws
Eat hot sauce
Master DOS
Ride a hoss
Paint our paws
Build with saws
Dress in gauze
Make oohs and aahs
Experiment with faux's
Or journey to Oz
In menopause?

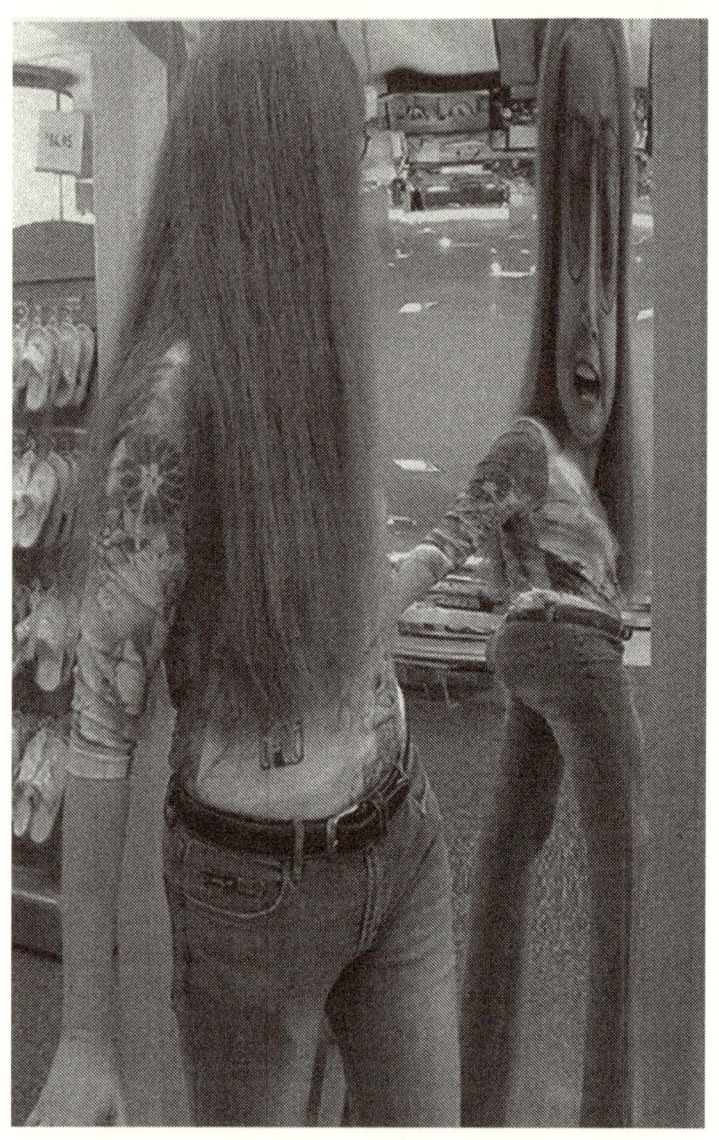

MIDLIFE THROUGH THE LOOKING GLASS

Check out your reflection
The 40 (50) something body
Hold in your gut
Stand up straight
Tighten those gluts
Add the push-up bra
Not bad, you think
If only I could hold my breath
Forever …
The mirror "you" would appear
Perfect, (well, it would be close)
But, don't put on those glasses
Oh nooooo!

QUARTERLY REPORT

I have a friend who tells me
That turning fifty
Is like entering into
The third quarter of
Your existence

I prefer to think of it
As my autumn, which
Evokes emotions attuned more
To a surrealist watercolor
Than to a bright acrylic canvas

Using either interpretation, find
That it is time to take notice
And make time to enjoy
This mortal realm
While you have vitality

I refuse to take
A negative stance
On this aging thing
We may not be able to beat it
But we can't just submit

We've got to harness
The power of our minds
Keep our bodies fit and lean
Feed our heads
And keep moving forward

There will be plenty of time
For bingo and mahjong
If that is what you choose
Let's try to stall the inevitable
What have you got to lose?

DIRECTORY ASSISTANCE

Sisters, I write to you today
My words formed from
The clarity
I now find within me

You can label these words
Bad poetry if you want, but
At least I have
The guts to reach out to you

I enlist your services in
Helping you to find you
To tap into your inner self, and
Find your true heart

Perhaps you won't receive
This wake-up call yet
Could it be your number is unlisted, or
Is your voice mail full, _**again?**_

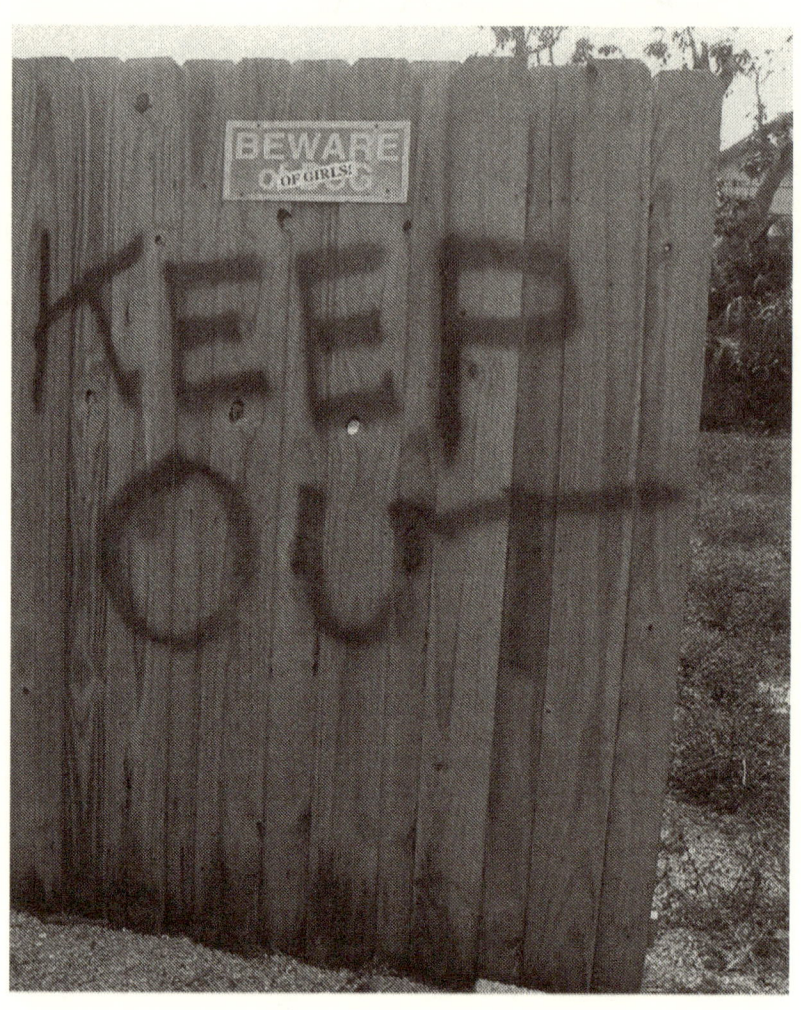

E-MAN-CIPATION

Is men-o-pause
A pause from men
Or time for a woman
To stop and breathe in
By taking men-tal routes
For themselves
Where men must *KEEP OUT*

In man-less awareness
May a woman turn inward
With introspection and assess
She must take inventory
Of her life and soul
Envision the future
Reach out for new goals

Until we ponder our fate
And unleash our lives
Our growth will stagnate
And never embrace "alive"
Though the wonder that we seek
And we very rarely find
Is hidden within the confines
Of our convoluted minds

EXERCISE IN MORPHOLOGY

Hush
Be very still
With eyes closed
And imagine you are
As a blank, white canvas
A page not yet written upon

Concentrate
On this image
Within your mind
Then use this background
To paint who you truly are
Using previous life as a guideline

Envision
The beautiful being
That you have within you
Sculpt and recreate yourself
With your dreams as the bones
Then flesh out the rest by sheer will

Live who you want to be!

REAL ESTATE

We are the architects of our lives
Every decision determines
The structure and shape
Of our fortresses

Sound thinking
Is the mortar and brick
Sense and sensibility
Are the cornerstones

Music, art, and creativity
Provide color and texture
While joy and happiness
Bring us comfort

Families and friends
Are our treasures
And love is the warm fire
In our heart of homes

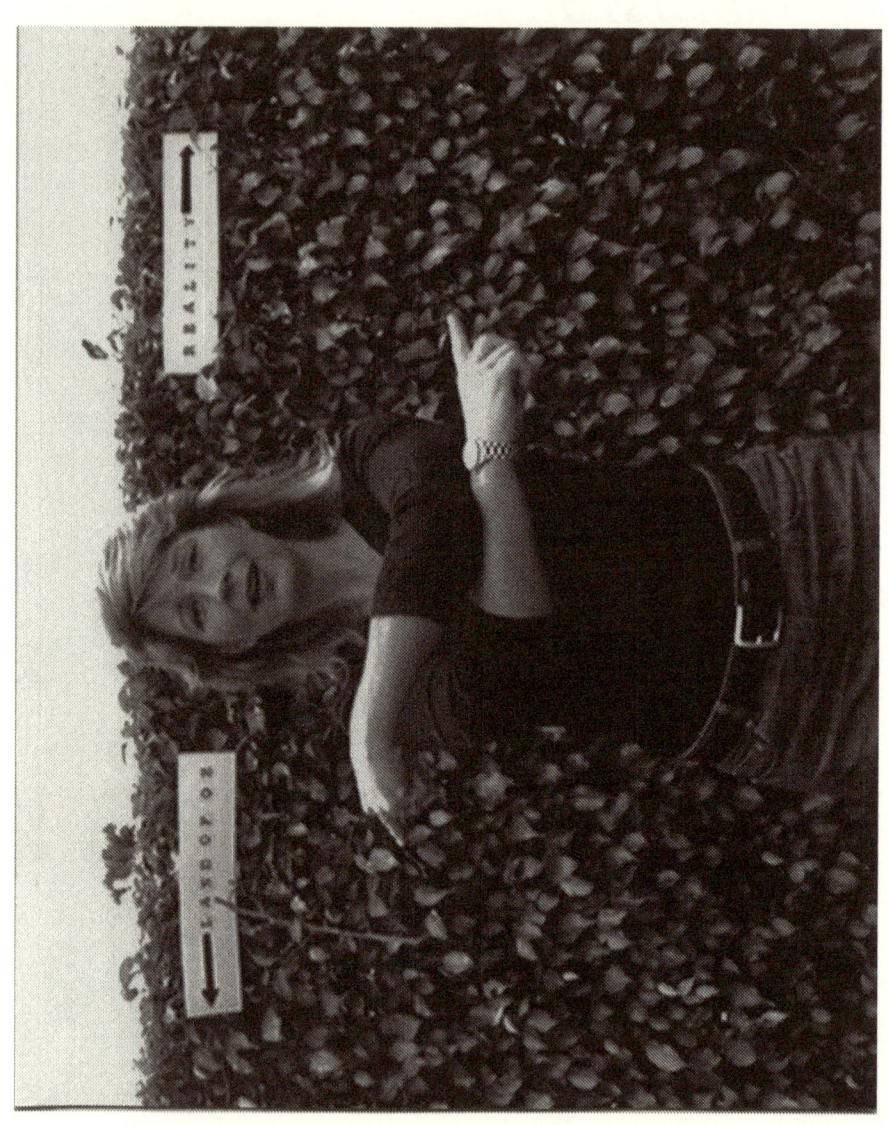

EXIST-STANCE

Meditate on this
If you do not make an effort
To live in the moment
You will not truly
Live

To always plan
For "Tomorrow Land"
Ignoring the boring minutia
You will never exist
In today

To chase after
What may be
One loses
The ability
To be

ABBI-NORMAL

How did I get to be "normal"
I spent my life being a square peg
Shy, then outrageous, or funny

I never wanted to go along for the ride
Always the individual
The rebel, resisting the status quo

I was a little late for Vietnam
Or I told myself, I would have protested
I was the flower child, moccasins and all

The 9 to 5 grind, and the pressures of
The working world have molded me
Rounding my prickly edges, somewhat

I have sensible clothes, tailored and proper
For work and the occasional event
Mainly, I have sturdy jeans and tees

I'm starting a renaissance of myself
Beginning with my closet
I am exorcising dull and boring
(Goodbye brown, hello purple!)

I've got my "cool" back
It was just misplaced, not forgotten
I may be a funky aging (?) hippie, but I have style
I love being this quietly outrageous person
One must be true to one's own self
This I accept, and applaud, loudly

Don't be a cookie cutter image of anyone
Find your true colors
And step into the unique garment of yourself!

SKIN DEEP

Worked into a frenzied froth of
Slick soap bubbles
Water beads up on
New, born-again
Baptized skin

Late afternoon light refracts
Through liquid droplets, as
Water flows across my chest, and
Dives downward, arcing
Into my belly-button, creating
a myriad of prismatic effects

As layers of grimy pollutants from
Daily stress, anger, and rudeness
(Man's inhumanity to woman)
Are scrubbed away; whirling
And spinning, exfoliated cells careen
Down the drain

I shed my workweek
False skin
My psyche feels resuscitated as
I evolve
Once more becoming
Human, for the weekend

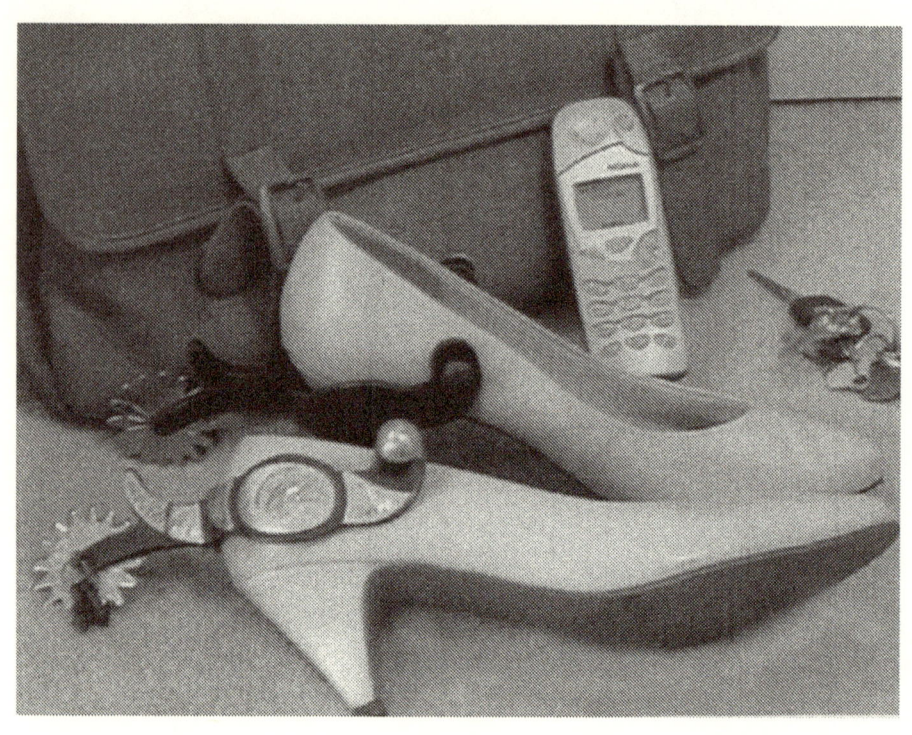

NEW FRONTIERS

I have to say that
The women I meet these days as
Peers, and otherwise
Are smart and savvy
They are really out there
Breaking up the male empire
And *enjoying* it

This sisterhood of women
Is such a positive force, and
Whether we realize it, or
Not, the truth is
Women are changing
Their worlds, and
It *is* apparent to them

Even if the rest of the planet cannot
See this alteration
It does not matter
It is our *own* perception that does
Women have visualized
A new reality, and made it theirs
They now operate within this new order

We are cowgirls of
The new frontier
Making and breaking up rules
We ride bareback into
Dangerous desert, canyons
(And boardrooms)
While twirling our palm pilots

When we wear our silver spurs
They haven't got a chance!

COCOON

Creating calm
In your life
Is as essential
To your existence
As oxygen

We have become
Hurried, harried
Hustling husks
We have forgotten
To breathe

Nullify the noise of
Modern life
Shipwreck yourself
On your island aerie
Nurture your native side

Unplug the phone
Cut off your cell
Become incommunicado
Turn off the tube
Acquiesce to quiet

Bask as bird song
Blends with the
Beating of your heart
Knowingly choose to be
A universe of one

Then, gratified and grounded
Will your authentic
Sated-self slip
Into your cocoon
Of silence

CATCH-22

When are you
Going to stop being
The victim?

It's not just your
Lot in life, you know
It is a cognizant choice.

You choose to believe
That you are inferior
You don't know your worth.

If you could see
The beautiful person that I see
You would fall in love with you.

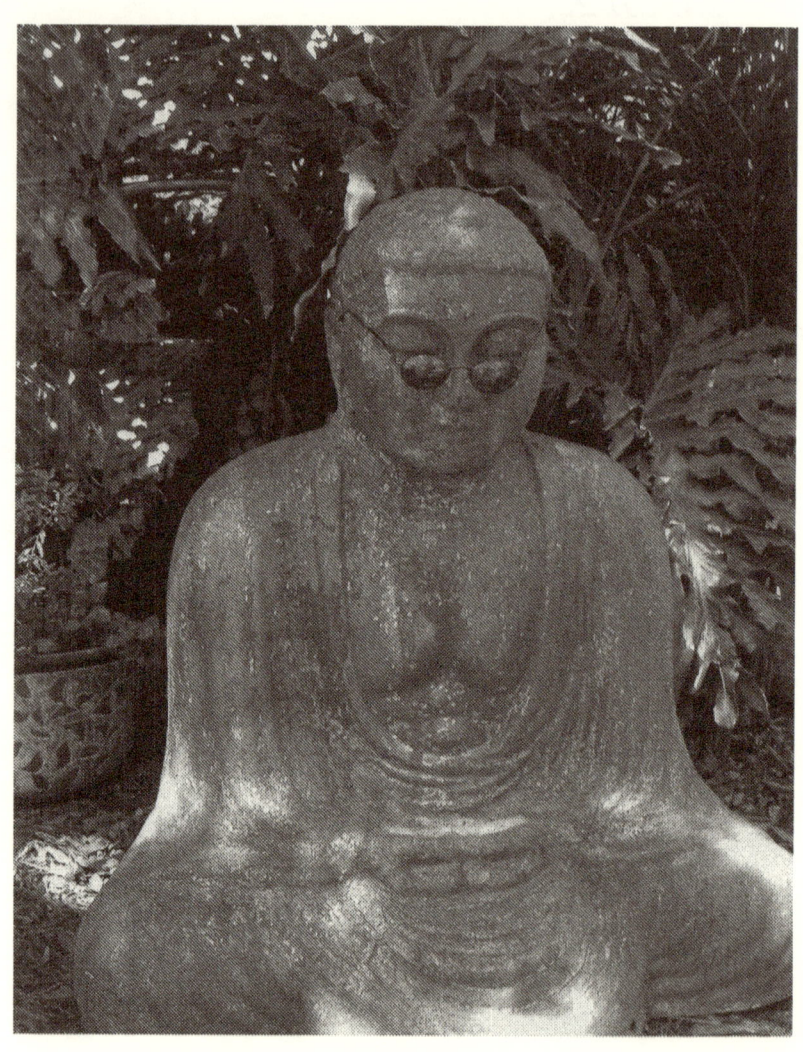

THE ZONE

While sequestered as a willing tenant in
Your self-made prison of busyness
Dream of ways you can be free

To give yourself the gift of
A precious few moments, no distractions
Lock out your outer "life" and meditate

Find that it is almost a new experience, as
You may have forgotten the sensation
Of pure awareness, and nothing else

So used to being the "amazing balancing act"
You have found it hard to stop doing and planning
And just become still

Discover that one can see so much clearer
When traveling at
The speed of now

OVERDRIVE

I cannot ignore
The erratic beating
Of my heart
Or the anxiety, the tightness
Surrounding my chest

Hormones abound, I feel the
Pressure in my skull increasing
An estrogen vice
Winding tighter still

Testosterone easily
Inflames my temper
My patience level
Is at low tide

I awake in the middle
Of the night with my steaming
Teakettle-head boiling
Ready to whistle

My body battles me to
Size up and up
I fight the fight daily
Or I will lose it

Calm and quiet beckon
Like a siren's song
I crave down time
Like an addict craves
Their addiction

START-LET

Tell me, did you get to be
What you wanted to be
When you grew up?

Did you get that dream job
Or, were you discovered
Like the mag-rags claimed you'd be?

Are you still that plain Jane
Working at the same old job
You told yourself was only temporary?

Things may not have moved on for you
Your life may be like stagnant water
With no flow, no progress, no future.

You could convince yourself
That it's not too late
And free yourself from your drab subsistence.

You might ask yourself, again
"What do I want to be, when I grow up?"
There is still time to find your purpose.

There is still time to find you.

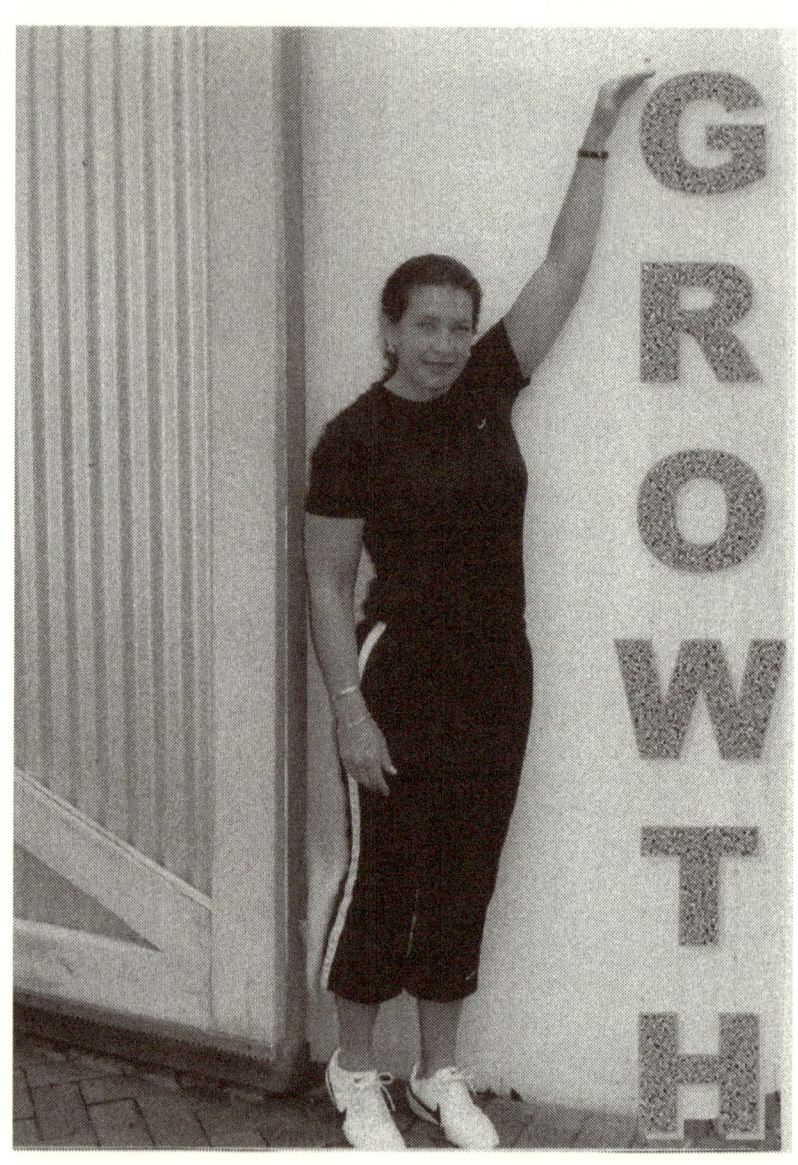

MEA CULPA

I have not come this far
In my life
Without making some mistakes
They are too numerous to list

If I were in a ten-step program
I would have to write letters
Apologizing for the harm
That I had caused others

We must accept the blame
For our own actions
Everything negative that happens to us
Is *not* our parents' fault

Facing up to life's consequences
Is a step on the road
To your self-recovery
Don't linger in failure; move forward!

CHANGLING

If you could be anywhere else
Traveling for parts unknown, or known
Where would you go?
Would you inform the "authorities"
Or just simply disappear …
Remaining a mystery to those left behind.
Such a romantic notion.

Think about it
You could live in a jungle
You Tarzana, (or Jane).
Or become a cowgirl
Riding and roping, sleeping under the stars.
How about becoming a film star
Like in Hollywood's heyday?

Don't forget your old friend fantasy
It can take you away
And help you plan your escape.
If you imagine and envision it
Your dream may be realized, as
In your mind's eye
It is conceived and delivered
With yourself as your own midwife.

Nothing happens in this world
Without your own support.
Either consciously or unconsciously
You let the stream of life pass by
Or, dive in as a willing participant.
Choose to struggle and rebuild
Or accept defeat, as the living dead
Do not lie down quietly; resurrect yourself!

STATE OF GRACE

I send this message
Out to you
Grasp it
Let it define you
Live it
Take it to heart

The revelation is that
This is the moment
The present, and
Nothing else exists
Be here
Seize the "now"

Be your bliss
And therefore
You shall be
Blessed

BY DESIGN

What is a breast?
It is, by design, in its simplest form
A source of nourishment
A literal "fountain of youth"

A breast is an ornament
Of the flesh, ascetically varied,
Rounded, pillowed, or arched
An achingly beautiful sculpture of nature

A breast is a haven
For comforting small humans
Or sheltering family and friends
With arms and bodies enfolded tightly, as in prayer

A breast can also give or receive
Pleasure, with our partners
As active participants
In the mating dance of life

A breast is the epitome of the heart
Of womankind, as with our breasts
We nurture, comfort, and love.
That is why we hold them so dear

Through breast cancer, women may
Lose these deeply personal pieces
Of their flesh, that share so much
And give succor to life

But, we must remember that
Women are the origin of strength
In this world, and with or
Without breasts, _**we are the same!**_

We will still nurture
We will still comfort
And we will still love
We will do this, by design

For Tina and all of her sisters

ONE TRIBE

Have you felt
With passing years
A more pressing
Need to connect
With other women
To share observations
And laughter
To offer advice
Or garner wisdom?
Do you feel drawn
As if by a magnetic force
To be with your own kind?

For these women
Are a tribe, *your* tribe.
No one else will ever
Understand your struggle
As they will.
Women are our *people*.
When we come together
We feel a oneness
A sisterhood united.
When we come together
We are at home.

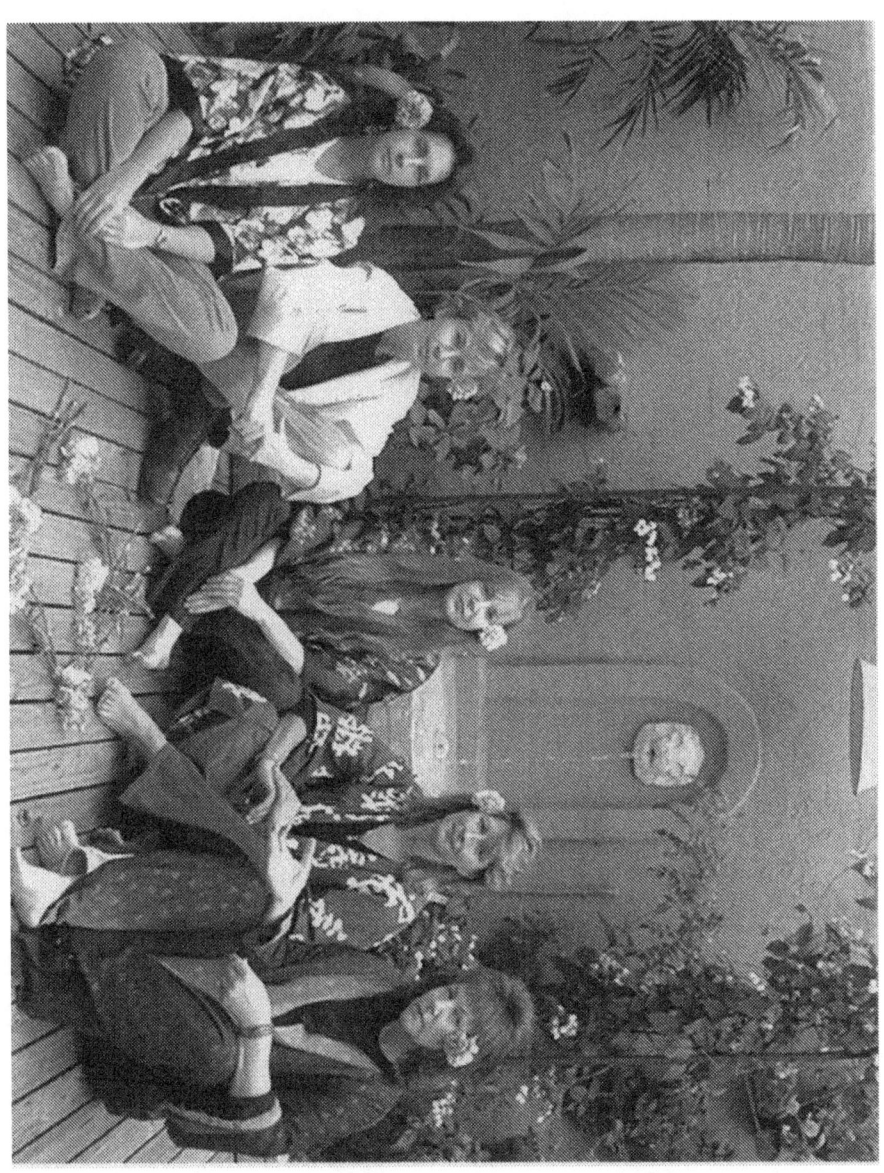

GIRLFRIEND

Friend of mine
There is purpose
In your sadness
You will find strength
In your struggle

There is no growth
Without discomfort
We do not learn
Without some pain
You will gain power
From this "education"

Persevere and pursue
Your karma
Your fate
Is in your own heart

WOMEN WHO SERVE

Daily, they bring me
The stories of their
Lives and loves
These tales speak
To me on a very
Personal level, as
These stories may
Evolve to include mine

These women tell me
Of lives spent
Taking care of everyone
Beginning with raising children
Encompassing perhaps twenty years
And of their being a helpmate
To their spouses, and doing
The never-ending household chores

But, these years of childrearing
Were closely followed with
The caretaking of these women's
Failing parents; a role reversal where
The parents seemed
To become the children
This was a difficult duty
But it was a duty done out of love

Lastly, the women spoke of
The deterioration of their spouses
Many of these women
Had no funds for outside help
And often were frail themselves
But they bravely served
At their spouses sides
And offered up their
Often-thankless support
Waging a war until the end

There are no purple hearts
For care-giving, and no memorials
This is the reality of women's lives
This may become your existence and mine
Please, learn by this lesson
This is our time; fly and be free!

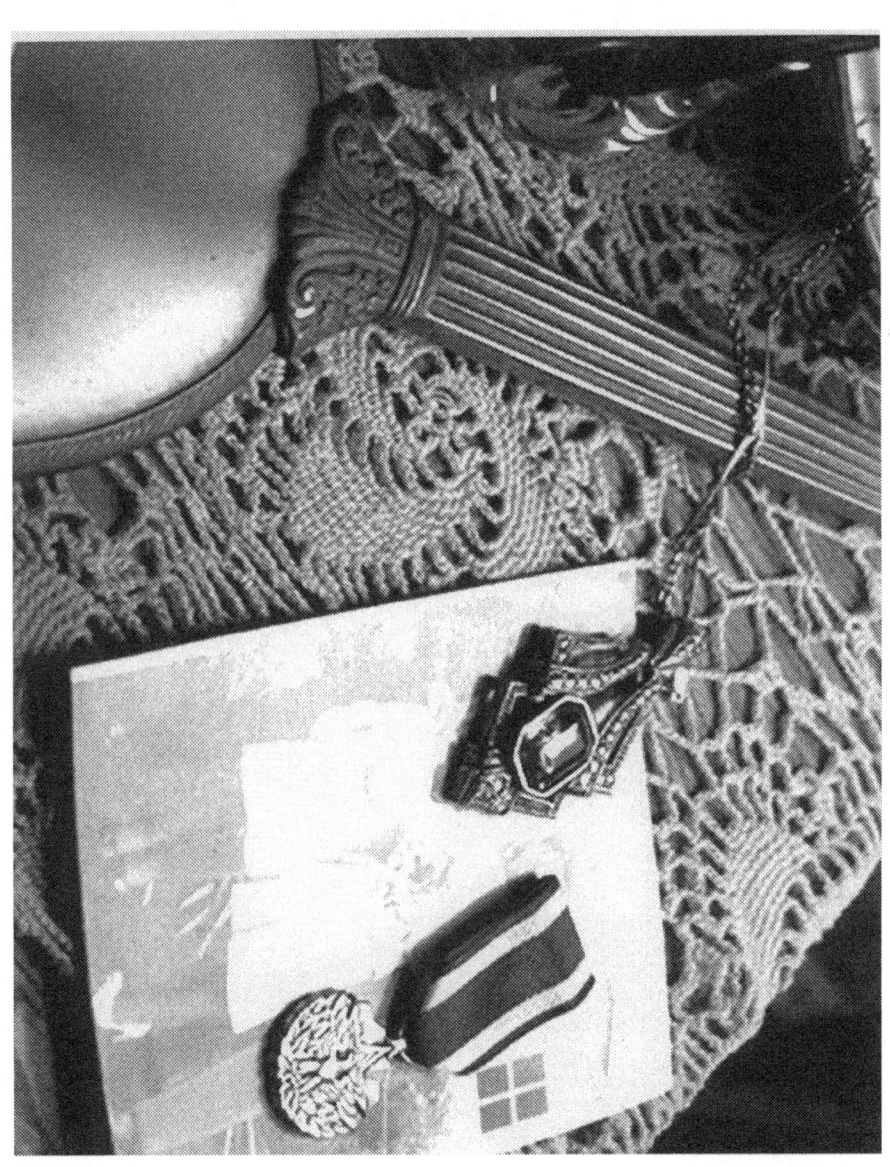

WATER RUNNING DOWNHILL!

I see my life
Like water running
Downhill, believing
Each precious droplet
Is a moment lost to me

For a time
My essence flowed
Calmly, evenly
In gentle
Creeks and rivulets

Then tiny streams
Became ever-widening rivers
Time cascaded, spiraled
Into whitewater rapids
Downward, rushing downward
Niagara Falls!

After the thundering crescendo, and
As the course of my being
Tapers, eventually becoming
An evaporating trickle
I will remember the deluge fondly
While coming to terms with
The imprint of my past life, knowing
My destiny awaits me like a dried-up river bed
Awaits the raging river

I see my life
Like water running downhill.
I see my life

DENIAL

Denial
Is not a river in Egypt
Or so I am told.

So get out and dance
To your music
Do it before you're too old!

ABOUT THE AUTHOR

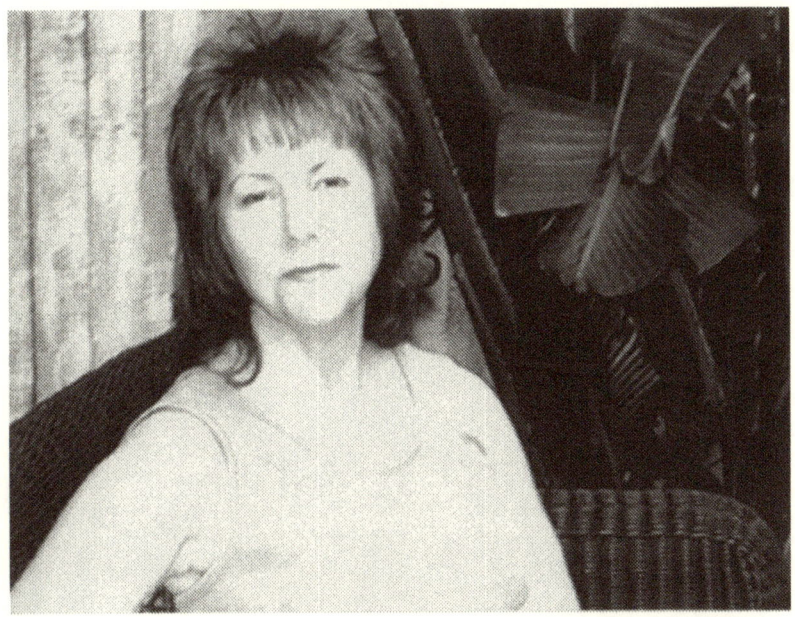

Joan Ellen Gage alternates between working in central Florida, and vacationing in western North Carolina. Her family includes her husband, Robert, and Belgian Tervuren, Magnolia. Joan has motivated and inspired dental hygiene patients for many years, while listening to their stories. This has spawned *Water Running Downhill!*, Joan's first publication.

978-0-595-42545-7
0-595-42545-3

www.ingramcontent.com/pod-product-compliance
Lightning Source LLC
Chambersburg PA
CBHW020358290526
45785CB00005B/2342